The Ultimate KETO Sweet Chaffle Cooking Guide

Amazing Sweet Chaffle Recipes For Beginners

Lily Sherman

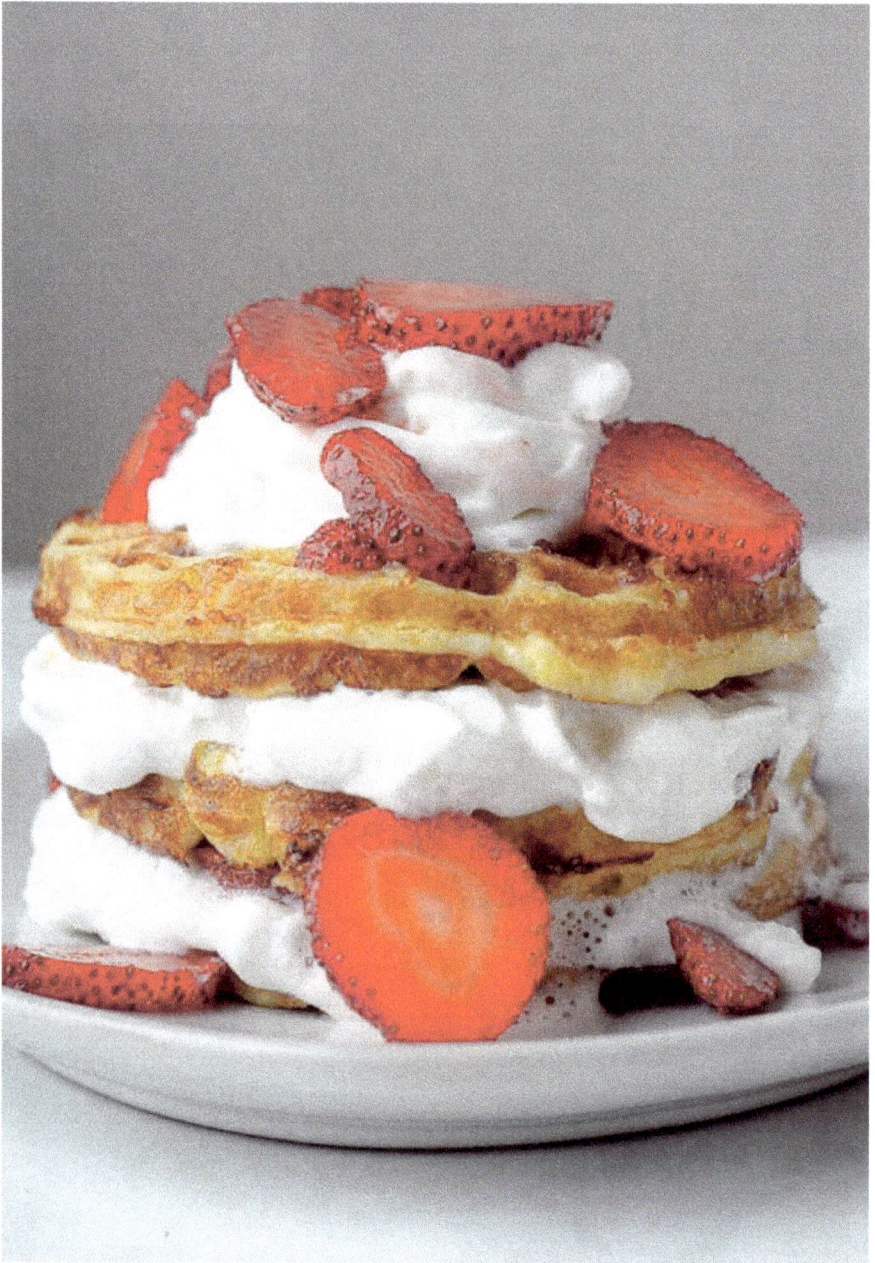

Table of contents

Chocolate Chip Chaffles

Cooking: 6 Minutes

Servings: 1

Ingredients

- 1 egg
- 1 tsp coconut flour
- 1 tsp sweetener
- ½ tsp vanilla extract
- ¼ cup heavy whipping cream, for serving
- ½ cup almond milk ricotta, finely shredded
- 2 tbsp sugar-free chocolate chips

Directions

1. Preheat now your mini waffle iron.
2. Mix now the egg, coconut flour, vanilla, and sweetener. Whisk together with a fork.
3. Stir in the almond milk ricotta.
4. Pour half of the batter into the waffle iron and dot with a pinch of chocolate chips.
5. Close the waffle iron and cook for minutes.

6. Repeat now with remaining batter.

7. Serve hot with the whipped cream.

Nutrition:

Calories: 304 Kcal, Fats: 16 g, Carbs: 7 g, Protein: 3 g

Pumpkin & Psyllium Husk Chaffles

Cooking: 16 Minutes

Servings: 4

Ingredients

- 2 organic eggs
- ½ cup mozzarella cheese, shredded
- 1 tbspn homemade pumpkin puree
- 2 teaspns Erythritol
- ½ teaspn psyllium husk powder
- 1/3 teaspn ground cinnamon
- Pinch of salt
- ½ teaspn organic vanilla extract

Directions

1. Preheat now a mini waffle iron and then grease it.
2. In a bowl, place all ingredients and beat until well combined.
3. Place ¼ of the mixture into Preheat waffle iron and cook for about 4 minutes or until golden brown.
4. Repeat now with the remaining mixture.

5. Serve warm.

Nutrition:

Net Carb: 0.6g, Fat: 2.8g, Saturated Fat: 1.1g, Carbohydrates: 0.8g, Dietary Fiber: 0.2g, Sugar: 0.4g, Protein: 3.9g

Keto Chocolate Fudge Chaffle

Cooking: 14 Minutes

Servings: 2

Ingredients

- 1 egg, beaten
- ¼ cup finely grated Gruyere cheese
- 2 tbsp unsweetened cocoa powder
- ¼ tsp baking powder
- ¼ tsp vanilla extract
- 2 tbsp erythritol
- 1 tsp almond flour
- 1 tsp heavy whipping cream
- A pinch of salt

Directions

1. Preheat now the waffle iron.
2. Add all the ingredients to a bowl and mix well.
3. Open the iron and add half of the mixture. Close and cook until golden brown and crispy, 7 minutes.
4. Remove now the chaffle onto a plate and make another with the remaining batter.

5. Cut each chaffle into wedges and serve after.

Nutrition:

Calories 173, Fats 13.08g, Carbs 3.98g, Net Carbs 2.28g, Protein 12.27g

Chaffled Brownie Sundae

Cooking: 30 Minutes

Servings: 4

Ingredients

For the chaffles:

- 2 eggs, beaten
- 1 tbsp unsweetened cocoa powder
- 1 tbsp erythritol
- 1 cup finely grated mozzarella cheese

For the topping:

- 3 tbsp unsweetened chocolate, chopped
- 3 tbsp unsalted butter
- ½ cup swerve sugar
- Low-carb ice cream for topping
- 1 cup whipped cream for topping
- 3 tbsp sugar-free caramel sauce

Directions

For the chaffles:

1. Preheat now the waffle iron.

2. Meanwhile, in a bowl, mix all the ingredients for the chaffles.

3. Open the iron, pour in a quarter of the mixture, cover, and cook until crispy, 7 minutes.

4. Remove now the chaffle onto a plate and make 3 more with the remaining batter.

5. Plate and set aside.

For the topping:

1. Meanwhile, melt the chocolate and butter in a medium saucepan with occasional stirring, 2 minutes.

To Servings:

1. Divide the chaffles into wedges and top with the ice cream, whipped cream, and swirl the chocolate sauce and caramel sauce on top.

2. Serve immediately.

Nutrition:

Calories 165, Fats 11.39g, Carbs 3.81g, Net Carbs 2.91g, Protein 79g

Krispy Kreme Copycat of Glazed Raspberry Jelly-Filled Donut

Cooking: 3 minutes

Preparation: 10 minutes

Ingredients

Chaffle:

- 1 egg
- 1/4 cup mozzarella cheese shredded
- 2 T cream cheese softened
- 1 T sweetener
- 1 T almond flour
- 1/2 tsp Baking Powder
- 20 drops glazed donut flavoring

Raspberry Jelly Filling:

- 1/4 cup raspberries
- 1 tsp chia seeds
- 1 tsp confectioners sweetener

Donut Glaze:

- 1 tsp powdered sweetener
- A few drops of water or heavy whipping cream

Directions

1. Mix everything to make the chaffles first.
2. Cook for about 2 1/2-3 minutes.

Make the Raspberry Jelly Filling:

3. Mix in a tiny pot on medium heat.
4. Gently mash raspberries.
5. Let cool.
6. Add between the layers of Chaffles.

Make the Donut Glaze:

7. Stir together in a tiny dish.
8. Drizzle on top Chaffle.

Keto Chocolate Twinkie Copycat Chaffle

Preparation: 5 minutes

Cooking: 12 minutes

Servings: 3

Ingredients

- 2 tbsps of butter (cooled)
- 2 oz. cream cheese softened
- Two large egg room temperature
- 1 teaspn of vanilla essence
- 1/4 cup Lacanto confectionery
- Pinch of pink salt
- 1/4 cup almond flour
- 2 tbsps coconut powder
- 2 tbsps cocoa powder
- 1 teaspn baking powder

Directions

1. Preheat now the Maker of Corndog.
2. Melt now the butter for a minute and let it cool.
3. In the butter, whisk the eggs until smooth.

4. Remove now sugar, cinnamon, sweetener and blend well.
5. Add flour of almond, flour of coconut, powder of cacao and baking powder.
6. Blend until well embedded.
7. Fill each well with ~2 tbsps of batter and spread evenly.
8. Close the lid and let it cooking for 4 minutes.
9. Lift from the rack and cool it down.

Nutrition:

Calories 202, Fat 6.6g, Carbs 2.9g, Protein 9.2g

Rice Krispie Treat Chaffle Copycat Recipe

Preparation: 15 minutes

Cooking: 5 minutes

Servings: 2

Ingredients

Chaffle Batter:

- 1 Large Egg room temp
- 2 oz. Cream Cheese softened
- 1/4 tsp Pure Vanilla Extract
- 2 tbs Lakanto Confectioners Sweetener
- 1 oz. Pork Rinds crushed
- 1 tsp Baking Powder

Marshmallow Frosting:

- 1/4 c. Heavy Whipping Cream
- 1/4 tsp Pure Vanilla Extract
- 1 tbs Lakanto Confectioners Sweetener
- 1/2 tsp Xanthan Gum

Directions

1. Plug in the mini waffle maker to Preheat now.
2. In a medium mixing bowl- Add egg, cream cheese, and vanilla.
3. Whisk until blended well.
4. Add sweetener, crushed pork rinds, and baking powder.
5. Mix well until well incorporated.
6. Sprinkle extra crushed pork rinds onto waffle maker (optional).
7. Then add about 1/4 scoop of batter over, sprinkle a bit more pork rinds.
8. Cook 3-4 min, then Remove now and cool on a wire rack.
9. Repeat for remaining batter.

Make the Marshmallow Frosting:

10. Whip the HWC, vanilla, and confectioners until thick and fluffy.
11. Slowly sprinkle over the xanthan gum and fold until well incorporated.
12. Spread frosting over chaffles and cut as desired, then refrigerate until set.
13. Enjoy cold or warm slightly in the microwave for 10 seconds.

Pumpkin Chaffle With Cream Cheese Glaze

Preparation: 5 minutes

Cooking: 5 minutes

Servings: 1

Ingredients

- 1 egg
- 1/2 cup Mozzarella cheese
- 1/2 tsp. pumpkin pie spice
- 1 tbsp. pumpkin

For the cream cheese frosting:

- 2 tbsp. cream cheese, softened at room temperature
- 2 tbsp. monkfruit
- 1/2 tsp. vanilla extract

Directions

1. Preheat now your waffle maker.
2. Whip the egg in a tiny bowl.
3. Add cheese, pumpkin, and pumpkin pie spice to the whipped egg and mix well.

4. Add half the batter to your waffle maker and cook for 3-4 minutes.

5. While waiting for the chaffle to cooking, combine all the ingredients for the frosting in another bowl. Continue mixing until a smooth and creamy consistency is reached. Feel free to add more butter if you prefer a buttery taste.

6. Allow the chaffle to cool before frosting it with cream cheese.

Nutrition:

25.4g Protein, 12.4g Carbohydrates, 1.2g Fat, 68gFiber, 63mg Cholesterol, 219mg Sodium, 408mg Potassium.

Blackberry Chaffles

Cooking: 8 Minutes

Servings: 2

Ingredients

- 1 organic egg, beaten
- 1/3 cup of Mozzarella cheese, shredded
- 1 teaspn cream cheese, softened
- 1 teaspn coconut flour
- ¼ teaspn organic baking powder
- ¾ teaspn powdered Erythritol
- ¼ teaspn ground cinnamon
- ¼ teaspn organic vanilla extract
- Pinch of salt
- 1 tbspn fresh blackberries

Directions

1. Preheat now a mini waffle iron and then grease it.
2. Place all ingredients except for blackberries and beat until well combined in a bowl.
3. Fold in the blackberries.

4. Place half of the mixture into preheated waffle iron and cook for about minutes or until golden brown.
5. Repeat now with the remaining mixture.
6. Serve warm.

Nutrition:

Calories: 121, Net Carb: 2g, Fat: 7.5g, Saturated Fat: 3.3g, Carbohydrates: 4.5g, Dietary Fiber: 1.8g, Sugar: 0.9g, Protein: 8.9g

Pumpkin Cream Cheese Chaffles

Cooking: 10 Minutes

Servings: 2

Ingredients

- 1 organic egg, beaten
- ½ cup Mozzarella cheese, shredded
- 1½ tbspn sugar-free pumpkin puree
- 2 teaspns heavy cream
- 1 teaspn cream cheese, softened
- 1 tbspn almond flour
- 1 tbspn Erythritol
- ½ teaspn pumpkin pie spice
- ½ teaspn organic baking powder
- 1 teaspn organic vanilla extract

Directions

1. Preheat now a mini waffle iron and then grease it.
2. In a bowl, place all ingredients and with a fork, Mix well until well combined.

3. Place half of the mixture into preheated waffle iron and cook for about 5 minutes or until golden brown.
4. Repeat now with the remaining mixture.
5. Serve warm.

Nutrition:

Calories: 110, Net Carb: 2.5g, Fat: 4.3g, Saturated Fat: 1g, Carbohydrates: 3.3g, Dietary Fiber: 0.8g, Sugar: 1g, Protein: 5.2g

Chaffles With Keto Ice Cream

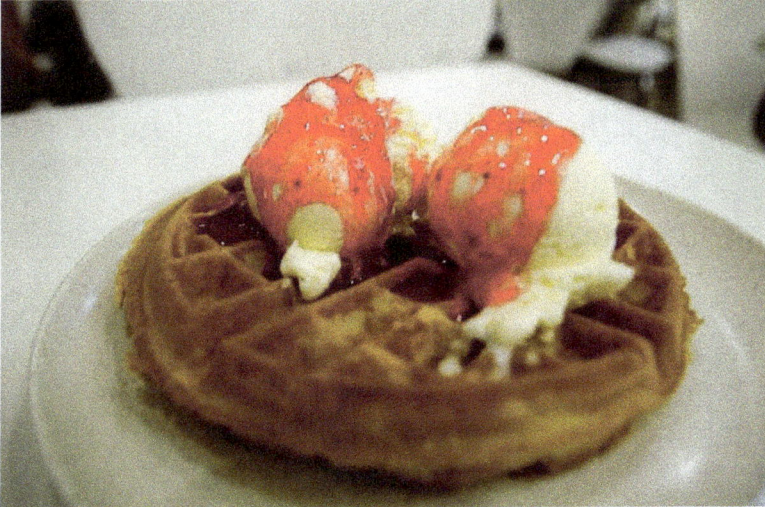

Cooking: 14 Minutes

Servings: 2

Ingredients

- 1 egg, beaten
- ½ cup finely grated mozzarella cheese
- ¼ cup almond flour
- 2 tbsp swerve confectioner's sugar
- 1/8 tsp xanthan gum
- Low-carb ice cream (flavor of your choice) for serving

Directions

1. Preheat now the waffle iron.
2. In a bowl, mix all the ingredients except the ice cream.
3. Open the iron and add half of the mixture. Close and cook until crispy, 7 minutes.
4. Transfer the chaffle to a plate and make second one with the remaining batter.
5. On each chaffle, add a scoop of low carb ice cream, fold into half-moons and enjoy.

Nutrition:

Calories 89, Fats 48g, Carbs 1.67g, Net Carbs 1.37g, Protein 5.91g

Vanilla Mozzarella Chaffles

Cooking: 12 Minutes

Servings: 2

Ingredients

- 1 organic egg, beaten
- 1 teaspn organic vanilla extract
- 1 tbspn almond flour
- 1 teaspn organic baking powder
- Pinch of ground cinnamon
- 1 cup Mozzarella cheese, shredded

Directions

1. Preheat now a mini waffle iron and then grease it.
2. Place the egg and vanilla extract and beat until well combined in a bowl.
3. Add the flour, baking powder and cinnamon and mix well.
4. Add the Mozzarella cheese and stir to combine.
5. Place half of the mixture into preheated waffle iron and cook for about 5-minutes or until golden brown.
6. Repeat now with the remaining mixture.

29

7. Serve warm.

Nutrition:

Calories: 103, Net Carb: 2.4g, Fat: 6.6g, Saturated Fat: 2.3g, Carbohydrates: 2, Dietary Fiber: 0.5g, Sugar: 0.6g, Protein: 6.8g

Cinnamon Pecan Chaffles

Cooking: 40 Minutes

Servings: 1

Ingredients

- 1 Tbsp butter
- 1 egg
- ½ tsp vanilla
- 2 Tbsp almond flour
- 1 Tbsp coconut flour
- ⅛ tsp baking powder
- 1 Tbsp monk fruit

For the crumble:

- ½ tsp cinnamon
- 1 Tbsp Melt butter
- 1 tsp monk fruit
- 1 Tbsp chopped pecans

Directions

1. Turn on waffle maker to heat and oil it with cooking spray.

2. Melt now butter in a bowl, then mix in the egg and vanilla.

3. Mix in remaining chaffle ingredients.

4. Combine crumble ingredients in a separate bowl.

5. Pour half of the chaffle mix into waffle maker. Top with half of crumble mixture.

6. Cook for 5 min, or until done.

7. Repeat now with the other half of the batter.

Nutrition:

Fat: 35 g, Protein: 10 g, Calories: 391

Chaffle Glazed with Raspberry

Cooking: 5 Minutes

Servings: 1

Ingredients

Donut Chaffle:

- 1 egg
- ¼ cup mozzarella cheese, shredded
- 2 tsp cream cheese, softened
- 1 tsp sweetener
- 1tsp almond flour
- ½ tsp baking powder
- 20 drops glazed donut flavoring

Raspberry Jelly Filling:

- ¼ cup raspberries
- 1 tsp chia seeds
- 1 tsp confectioners sweetener

Donut Glaze:

- 1 tsp powdered sweetener
- Heavy whipping cream

Directions

1. Spray your waffle maker with cooking oil and add the batter mixture into your waffle maker.
2. Cook for 3 minutes and set aside.

Raspberry Jelly Filling:

3. Mix all the
4. Place in a pot and heat on medium.
5. Gently mash the raspberries and set aside to cool.

Donut Glaze:

6. Stir together the ingredients

Assembling:

7. Lay your chaffles on a plate and add the layers' fillings mixture.
8. Drizzle the glaze on top and enjoy.

Nutrition:

Calories: 188 Kcal , Fats: 23 g, Carbs: 12 g, Protein: 17 g

Brownie Chaffle

Preparation: 5 minutes

Cooking: 3 minutes

Servings: 2

Ingredients

- 1 Egg Whisked
- 1/3 cup of Mozzarella cheese Shredded
- 1 ½ tbsp. Cocoa Powder Dutch Processed
- 1 tbsp. Almond Flour
- 1 tbsp. Monkfruit Sweetener
- 1/4 tsp. Vanilla extract
- 1/4 tsp. Baking Powder
- Pinch of Salt
- 2 tsp. Heavy Cream

Directions

1. First step as always is to preheat your mini waffle iron.
2. Next, whisk the egg. Add the dry ingredients. Then add the cheese in a bowl. Then you pour 1/3 of the batter on the waffle iron.

3. Allow to cooking for 3 minutes or until steam stops coming out of the waffle iron.

4. Serve with your favorite low carb toppings.

Nutrition:

Calories 273, Fat 8.4 g, Saturated Fat 2.3 g, Carbohydrate 16.7 g, Dietary Fiber 2.2 g, Protein 30.7 g, Cholesterol 78 mg, Sugars 3.5 g, Sodium 1501 mg, Potassium 633 mg

Banana Foster Chaffle

Preparation: 10 minutes

Cooking: 20 minutes

Servings: 4 large chaffles

Ingredients

<u>For Chaffle:</u>

- 1/8 teaspn cinnamon
- ½ teaspn banana extract, unsweetened
- 4 teaspns swerve sweetener
- 1 cup / 225 grams cream cheese, softened
- ½ teaspn vanilla extract, unsweetened
- 8 eggs, at room temperature

<u>For Syrup:</u>

- 20 drops of banana extract, unsweetened
- 8 teaspns swerve sweetener
- 20 drops of caramel extract, unsweetened
- drops of rum extract, unsweetened
- 8 tbsps unsalted butter
- 1/8 teaspn cinnamon

Directions:

1. Take a non-stick waffle iron, plug it in, select the medium or medium-high heat setting and let it Preheat now until ready to use; it could also be indicated with an indicator light changing its color.

2. Meanwhile, the batter for chaffle and this, take a large bowl, crack eggs in it, add sweetener, cream cheese, and all the extracts and then mix with an electric mixer until smooth, let the batter stand for 5 minutes.

3. Use a spoon to pour one-fourth of the prepared batter into the heated waffle iron in a spiral direction, starting from the edges, then shut the lid and cooking for 5 minutes or more until solid and nicely browned; the cooked waffle will look like a cake.

4. When done, transfer chaffles to a plate with a silicone spatula, repeat now with the remaining batter and let chaffles stand for some time until crispy.

5. Meanwhile, the syrup and this take a tiny heatproof bowl, add butter in it, and microwave at high heat setting for 15 seconds until it melt.

6. Then add remaining ingredients for the syrup and Mix well until combined.

7. Drizzle syrup over chaffles and then serve.

Nutrition:

Calories 440, Fat 6 g, Saturated fat 0 g, Carbohydrates 33 g, Fiber 4 g, Protein 30 g, Cholesterol 0 mg, Sugars 1 g, Sodium 220 mg, Potassium 135 mg

Oreo Keto Chaffles

Cooking: 5 Minutes

Servings: 2

Ingredients

- 1 egg
- 1½ Tbsp unsweetened cocoa
- 2 Tbsp lakanto monk fruit, or choice of sweetener
- 1 Tbsp heavy cream
- 1 tsp coconut flour
- ½ tsp baking powder
- ½ tsp vanilla

For the cheese cream:

- 1 Tbsp lakanto powdered sweetener
- 2 Tbsp softened cream cheese
- ¼ tsp vanilla

Directions

1. Turn on waffle maker to heat and oil it with cooking spray.
2. Combine all chaffle ingredients in a tiny bowl.

3. Pour one half of the chaffle mixture into waffle maker. Cook for 5 minutes.
4. Remove now and repeat with the second half of the mixture. Let chaffles sit for 2-3 to crisp up.
5. Combine all cream ingredients and spread on chaffle when they have cooled to room temperature.

Nutrition:

Carbs: 3 g ;Fat: 4 g ;Protein: 7 g ;Calories:

Cinnamon Sugar Chaffles

Cooking: 12 Minutes

Servings: 2

Ingredients

- 2 eggs
- 1 cup Mozzarella cheese, shredded
- 2 tbsp blanched almond flour
- ½ tbsp butter, Melt
- 2 tbsp Erythritol
- ½ tsp cinnamon
- ½ tsp vanilla extract
- ½ tsp psyllium husk powder, optional
- ¼ tsp baking powder, optional
- 1 tbsp Melt butter, for topping
- ¼ cup Erythritol, for topping
- ¾ tsp cinnamon, for topping

Directions

- Pour enough batter into your waffle maker and cook for 4 minutes.

- Once it's cooked, carefully remove the chaffle and set aside.
- Repeat now with the remaining batter the same steps.
- Stir together the cinnamon and erythritol.
- Finish by brushing your chaffles with the melt butter and then sprinkle with cinnamon sugar.

Nutrition:

Calories: 208 Kcal, Fats: 16 g, Carbs: 4 g, Protein: 11 g

Cream Cheese Chaffles

Cooking: 8 Minutes

Servings: 2

Ingredients

- 2 teaspns coconut flour
- 3 teaspns Erythritol
- ¼ teaspn organic baking powder
- 1 organic egg, beaten
- 1 ounce of cream cheese, softened
- ½ teaspn organic vanilla extract

Directions

1. Preheat now a mini waffle iron and then grease it.
2. Place flour, Erythritol, baking powder, and mix well in a bowl.
3. Add the egg, cream cheese and vanilla extract and beat until well combined.
4. Place half of the mixture into the preheated waffle iron and cook for about 3-minutes or until golden brown.

5. Repeat now with the remaining mixture.

6. Serve warm.

Nutrition:

Calories: 95, Net Carb: 1.6g, Fat: 4g, Saturated Fat: 4g, Carbohydrates: 2.6g, Dietary Fiber: 1g, Sugar: 0.3g, Protein: 4.2g

Mozzarella & Butter Chaffles

Cooking: 8 Minutes

Servings: 2

Ingredients

- 1 large organic egg, beaten
- ¾ cup Mozzarella cheese, shredded
- ½ tbspn unsalted butter, Melt
- 2 tbsps blanched almond flour
- 2 tbsps Erythritol
- ½ teaspn ground cinnamon
- ½ teaspn Psyllium husk powder
- ¼ teaspn organic baking powder
- ½ teaspn organic vanilla extract

Directions

- Preheat now a waffle iron and then grease it.
- In a bowl, place all ingredients and with a fork, mix until well combined.

- Place half of the mixture into the preheated waffle iron and cook for about 5 minutes or until golden brown.
- Repeat now with the remaining mixture.
- Serve warm.

Nutrition:

Calories: 140, Net Carb: 1.9g, Fat: 10g, Saturated Fat: 4g, Carbohydrates: 3g, Dietary Fiber: 1.1g, Sugar: 0.3g, Protein: 7.8g

Pumpkin Pecan Chaffles

Cooking: 10 Minutes

Servings: 2

Ingredients

- 1 egg
- ½ cup mozzarella cheese grated
- 1 Tbsp pumpkin puree
- ½ tsp pumpkin spice
- 1 tsp erythritol low carb sweetener
- 2 Tbsp almond flour
- 2 Tbsp pecans, toasted chopped
- 1 cup heavy whipped cream
- ¼ cup low carb caramel sauce

Directions

1. Turn on waffle maker to heat and oil it with cooking spray.
2. In a bowl, beat egg.
3. Mix in mozzarella, pumpkin, flour, pumpkin spice, and erythritol.

4. Stir in pecan pieces.
5. Spoon one half of the batter into waffle maker and spread evenly.
6. Close and cook for 5 minutes.
7. Remove now cooked waffles to a plate.
8. Repeat now with remaining batter.
9. Serve with pecans, whipped cream, and low carb caramel sauce.

Nutrition:

Carbs: 4 g, Fat: 17 g, Protein: 11 g, Calories: 210

Chocolate Cream Chaffles

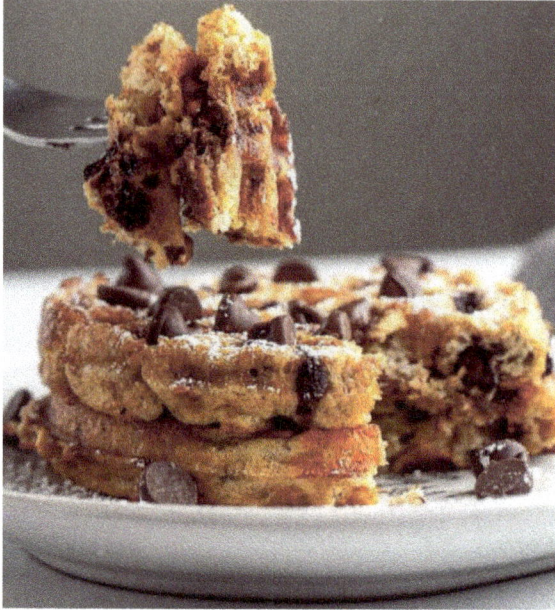

Cooking: 10 Minutes

Servings: 2

Ingredients

- 1 organic egg
- 1½ tbsps cacao powder
- 2 tbsps Erythritol
- 1 tbspn heavy cream
- 1 teaspn coconut flour

- ½ teaspn organic baking powder
- ½ teaspn organic vanilla extract
- ½ teaspn powdered Erythritol

Directions

- Preheat now a mini waffle iron and then grease it.
- Place all ingredients except the powdered Erythritol and beat until well combined in a bowl.
- Place half of the mixture into the preheated waffle iron and cook for about 5 minutes or until golden brown.
- Repeat now with the remaining mixture.
- Serve warm with the sprinkling of powdered Erythritol.

Nutrition:

Net Carb: 2.1g, Fat: 5.9g, Saturated Fat: 3g, Carbohydrates: 3.8g, Dietary Fiber: 1.7g, Sugar: 0.3g, Protein: 3.8g

Blueberry Cinnamon Chaffles

Cooking: 10 Minutes

Servings: 3

Ingredients

- 1 cup shredded mozzarella cheese
- 3 Tbsp almond flour
- 2 eggs
- 2 tsp Swerve or granulated sweetener of choice
- 1 tsp cinnamon
- ½ tsp baking powder
- ½ cup fresh blueberries
- ½ tsp of powdered Swerve

Directions

1. Turn on waffle maker to heat and oil it with cooking spray.
2. Mix eggs, flour, mozzarella, cinnamon, vanilla extract, sweetener, and baking powder in a bowl until well combined.
3. Add in blueberries.

4. Pour ¼ batter into each waffle mold.

5. Close and cook for 8 minutes.

6. If it's crispy and your waffle maker opens without pulling the

7. chaffles apart, the chaffle is ready. If not, close and cook for 1-2 minutes more.

8. Serve with favorite topping and more blueberries.

Nutrition:

Carbs: 9 g, Fat: 12 g, Protein: 13 g, Calories: 193

Strawberry Shortcake Chaffles

Cooking: 25 Minutes

Servings: 1

Ingredients

For the Batter:

- 1 egg
- ¼ cup mozzarella cheese
- 1 Tbsp cream cheese
- ¼ tsp baking powder
- 2 strawberries, sliced
- 1 tsp strawberry extract

For the glaze:

- 1 Tbsp cream cheese
- ¼ tsp strawberry extract
- 1 Tbsp monk fruit confectioners blend

For the whipped cream:

- 1 cup heavy whipping cream
- 1 tsp vanilla
- 1 Tbsp monk fruit

Directions

1. Turn on waffle maker to heat and oil it with cooking spray.
2. Beat egg in a tiny bowl.
3. Add remaining batter components.
4. Divide the mixture in half.
5. Cook one half of the batter in a waffle maker for 4 min, or until golden brown.
6. Repeat now with remaining batter
7. Mix all glaze ingredients and spread over each warm chaffle.
8. Mix all whipped cream ingredients and whip until it starts to form peaks.
9. Top each waffle with whipped cream and strawberries.

Nutrition:

Carbs: 5 g, Fat: 14 g, Protein: 12 g, Calories: 218

Vanilla Chaffle

Cooking: 8 Minutes

Servings: 2

Ingredients

- 2 tbsp butter, softened
- 2 oz cream cheese, softened
- 2 eggs
- ¼ cup almond flour
- 2 tbsp coconut flour
- 1 tsp baking powder
- 1 tsp vanilla extract
- ¼ cup confectioners
- Pinch of pink salt

Directions

1. Preheat now your waffle maker and spray with non-stick cooking spray.
2. Melt now the butter and set aside for a minute to cool.

3. Add the eggs into the melted butter and whisk until creamy.
4. Pour in the sweetener, vanilla, extract, and salt. Blend properly.
5. Next add the coconut flour, almond flour, and baking powder. Mix well.
6. Pour into your waffle maker and cook for 4 minutes.
7. Repeat the process with the remaining batter.
8. Remove now and set aside to cool.
9. Enjoy.

Nutrition:

Calories: 202 Kcal, Fats: 27 g, Carbs: 9 g, Protein: 23 g

Banana Nut Chaffle

Cooking: 10 Minutes

Servings: 1

Ingredients

- 1 egg
- 1 Tbsp cream cheese, softened and room temp
- 1 Tbsp sugar-free cheesecake pudding
- ½ cup mozzarella cheese
- 1 Tbsp monk fruit confectioners sweetener
- ¼ tsp vanilla extract
- ¼ tsp banana extract
- toppings of choice

Directions

1. Turn on waffle maker to heat and oil it with cooking spray.
2. Beat egg in a tiny bowl.
3. Add remaining ingredients and mix well until well incorporated.

4. Add one half of the batter to waffle maker and cook for min, until golden brown.
5. Remove now chaffle and add the other half of the batter.
6. Top with your optional toppings and serve warm!

Nutrition:

Carbs: 2 g, Fat: g, Protein: 8 g, Calories: 119

Chocolaty Chips Pumpkin Chaffles

Cooking: 12 Minutes

Servings: 3

Ingredients

- 1 organic egg
- 4 teaspns homemade pumpkin puree
- ½ cup Mozzarella cheese, shredded
- 1 tbspn almond flour
- 2 tbsps granulated Erythritol
- ¼ teaspn pumpkin pie spice
- 4 teaspns 70% dark chocolate chips

Directions

1. In a bowl, place the egg and pumpkin puree and mix well.
2. Add the remaining ingredients except for chocolate chips and Mix well until well combined.
3. Gently, fold in the chocolate chips and lemon zest.

4. Place 1/3 of the mixture into the preheated waffle iron and cook for about minutes or until golden brown.
5. Repeat now with the remaining mixture.
6. Serve warm.

Nutrition:

Net Carb: 1.9g, Fat: 7.1g, Saturated Fat: 3.3g, Carbohydrates: 1.4g, Dietary Fiber: 2.6g, Sugar: 0.4g, Protein: 4.2g

Whipping Cream Pumpkin Chaffles

Cooking: 12 Minutes

Servings: 4

Ingredients

- 2 organic eggs
- 2 tbsps homemade pumpkin puree
- 2 tbsps heavy whipping cream
- 1 tbspn coconut flour
- 1 tbspn Erythritol
- 1 teaspn pumpkin pie spice
- ½ teaspn organic baking powder
- ½ teaspn organic vanilla extract
- Pinch of salt
- ½ cup Mozzarella cheese, shredded

Directions

- Preheat now a mini waffle iron and then grease it.
- Place all the ingredients except Mozzarella cheese and beat until well combined in a bowl.
- Add the Mozzarella cheese and stir to combine.

- Place half of the mixture into the preheated waffle iron and cook for about 6 minutes or until golden brown.
- Repeat now with the remaining mixture.
- Serve warm.

Nutrition:

Calories: 81, Net Carb: 2.1g, Fat: 5.9g, Saturated Fat: 3g, Carbohydrates: 3.1g, Dietary Fiber: 1g, Sugar: 0.5g, Protein: 4.3g

Chocolate Vanilla Chaffles

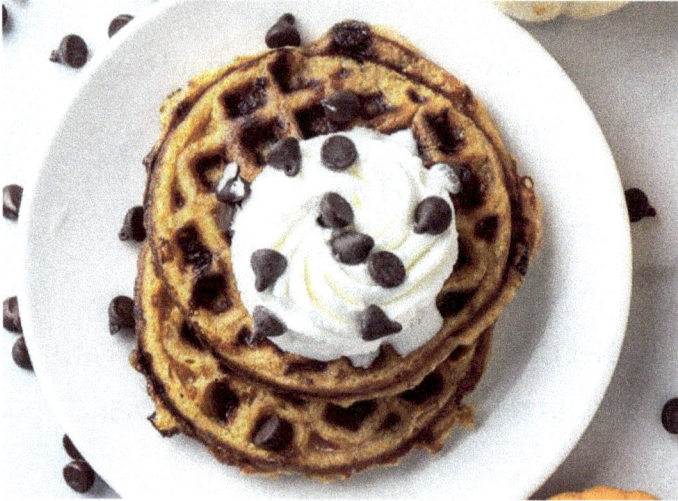

Cooking: 5 Minutes

Servings: 2

Ingredients

- ½ cup shredded mozzarella cheese
- 1 egg
- 1 Tbsp granulated sweetener
- 1 tsp vanilla extract
- 1 Tbsp sugar-free chocolate chips
- 2 Tbsp almond meal/flour

Directions

- Turn on waffle maker to heat and oil it with cooking spray.
- Mix all components in a bowl until combined.
- Pour half of the batter into waffle maker.
- Cook for 2-min, then remove now and repeat with remaining batter.
- Top with more chips and favorite toppings.

Nutrition:

Carbs: 23 g, Fat: 3 g, Protein: 4 g, Calories: 134

Churro Waffles

Cooking: 10 Minutes

Servings: 1

Ingredients

- 1 tbsp coconut cream
- 1 egg
- 6 tbsp almond flour
- ¼ tsp xanthan gum
- ½ tsp cinnamon
- 2 tbsp keto brown sugar

Coating:

- 2 tbsp butter, Melted
- 1 tbsp keto brown sugar
- Warm up your waffle maker.

Directions

1. Pour half of the batter to the waffle pan and cook for 5 minutes.
2. Carefully remove now the cooked waffle and repeat the steps with the remaining batter.

3. Allow the chaffles to cool and spread with the melted butter and top with the brown sugar.

4. Enjoy.

Nutrition:

Calories: 178 Kcal, Fats: 15.7 g, Carbs: 3.9 g, Protein: 2 g

Chocolate Chips Lemon Chaffles

Cooking: 8 Minutes

Servings: 4

Ingredients

- 2 organic eggs
- ½ cup Mozzarella cheese, shredded
- ¾ teaspn organic lemon extract
- ½ teaspn organic vanilla extract
- 2 teaspns Erythritol
- ½ teaspn psyllium husk powder
- Pinch of salt
- 1 tbspn 70% dark chocolate chips
- ¼ teaspn lemon zest, grated finely

Directions

- Preheat now a mini waffle iron and then grease it.
- Place all ingredients except chocolate chips and lemon zest and beat until well combined in a bowl.
- Gently, fold in the chocolate chips and lemon zest.

- Place ¼ of the mixture into the preheated waffle iron and cook for about minutes or until golden brown.
- Repeat now with the remaining mixture.
- Serve warm.

Nutrition:

Net Carb: 1g, Fat: 4.8g, Saturated Fat: 2.3g, Carbohydrates: 1.5g, Dietary Fiber: 0.5g, Sugar: 0.3g, Protein: 4.3g

Chocolate Sandwich Chaffles

Cooking: 10 minutes

Servings: 2

Ingredients

Chaffles:

- 1 organic egg, beaten
- 1 ounce of cream cheese, softened
- 2 tbsps almond flour
- 1 tbspn cacao powder
- 2 teaspns erythritol
- 1 teaspn organic vanilla extract

Filling:

- 2 tbsps cream cheese, softened
- 2 tbsps erythritol
- 1/2 tbspn cacao powder
- 1/4 teaspn organic vanilla extract

Directions

1. Preheat now a mini waffle iron and then grease it.

2. For chaffles: In a bowl, put all ingredients and with a fork, mix until well combined.

3. Place half of the mixture into preheated waffle iron and cook for about 3-5 minutes.

4. Repeat now with the remaining mixture.

5. Meanwhile, for filling: In a bowl, put all ingredients and with a hand mixer, beat until well combined.

6. Serve each chaffle with chocolate mixture.

Nutrition:

Calories 192, Total Fat 16 g, Saturated Fat 7.6 g, Cholesterol 113 mg, Sodium 115 mg, Total Carbs 4.4 g, Fiber 1.9 g, Sugar 0.8 g, Protein 5.7 g

Carrot Chaffles

Cooking: 18 Minutes

Servings: 6

Ingredients

- ¾ cup almond flour
- 1 tbspn walnuts, chopped
- 2 tbsps powdered Erythritol
- 1 teaspn organic baking powder
- ½ teaspn ground cinnamon
- ½ teaspn pumpkin pie spice
- 1 organic egg, beaten
- 2 tbsps heavy whipping cream
- 2 tbsps butter, Melted
- ½ cup carrot, peeled and shredded

Directions

1. Preheat now a mini waffle iron and then grease it.
2. Place the flour, walnut, Erythritol, cinnamon, baking powder and spices and mix well in a bowl.

3. Add the egg, heavy whipping cream and butter and mix well until combined.
4. Gently, fold in the carrot.
5. Add about 3 tbsps of the mixture into preheated waffle iron and cook for about 2½-3 minutes or until golden brown.
6. Repeat now with the remaining mixture.
7. Serve warm.

Nutrition:

Calories: 165, Net Carb: 2.4g, Fat: 14.7g, Saturated Fat: 4.4g, Carbohydrates: 4.4g, Dietary Fiber: 2g, Sugar: 1g, Protein: 1.5g

Chocolate Peanut Butter Chaffles

Cooking: 8 Minutes

Servings: 2

Ingredients

- 1 organic egg, beaten
- ¼ cup mozzarella cheese, shredded
- 2 tbsps creamy peanut butter
- 1 tbspn almond flour
- 1 tbspn granulated erythritol
- 1 teaspn organic vanilla extract
- 1 tbspn 70% dark chocolate chips

Directions

1. Preheat now a mini waffle iron and then grease it.
2. In a bowl, add all ingredients except chocolate and beat until well combined.Gently, fold in the chocolate chips.
3. Place half of the mixture into preheated waffle iron and cook for about 4 minutes.
4. Repeat now with the remaining mixture.

5. Serve warm.

Nutrition:

Calories 214, Net Carbs 4.1 g, Total Fat 18 g, Saturated Fat 5.4 g, Cholesterol 84 mg, Sodium 128 mg, Total Carbs 6.4 g, Fiber 2.3 g, Sugar 2.1 g, Protein 8.8 g

Berries Chaffles

Cooking: 10 Minutes

Servings: 2

Ingredients

- 1 organic egg
- 1 teaspn organic vanilla extract
- 1 tbspn of almond flour
- 1 teaspn organic baking powder
- Pinch of ground cinnamon
- 1 cup Mozzarella cheese, shredded
- 2 tbsps fresh blueberries
- 2 tbsps fresh blackberries

Directions

1. Preheat now a waffle iron and then grease it.
2. In a bowl, place thee egg and vanilla extract and beat well.
3. Add the flour, baking powder and cinnamon and mix well.
4. Add the Mozzarella cheese and mix well until just combined.

5. Gently, fold in the berries.

6. Place half of the mixture into preheated waffle iron and cook for about 4-5 minutes or until golden brown.

7. Repeat now with the remaining mixture.

8. Serve warm.

Nutrition:

Calories: 112, Net Carb: 3.8g, Fat: 6.7g, Saturated Fat: 2.3g, Carbohydrates: 5g, Dietary Fiber: 1.2g, Sugar: 1g, Protein: 7g

Cinnamon Swirl Chaffles

Cooking: 12 Minutes

Servings: 3

Ingredients

<u>For Chaffles:</u>

- 1 organic egg
- ½ cup Mozzarella cheese, shredded
- 1 tbspn almond flour
- ¼ teaspn organic baking powder
- 1 teaspn granulated Erythritol
- 1 teaspn ground cinnamon

<u>For Topping:</u>

- 1 tbspn butter
- 1 teaspn ground cinnamon
- 2 teaspns powdered Erythritol

Directions

1. Preheat now a waffle iron and then grease it.
2. For chaffles: in a bowl, place all ingredients and mix well until well combined.

3. For topping: in a tiny microwave-safe bowl, place all ingredients and microwave for about 15 seconds.
4. Remove now from microwave and mix well.
5. Place 1/3 of the chaffles mixture into preheated waffle iron.
6. Top with 1/3 of the butter mixture and with a skewer, gently swirl into the chaffles mixture.
7. Cook for about 3-4 minutes or until golden brown.
8. Repeat now with the remaining chaffles and topping mixture.
9. Serve warm.

Nutrition:

Calories: 87, Net Carb: 1g, Fat: 7.4g, Saturated Fat: 3.5g, Carbohydrates: 2.1g, Dietary Fiber: 1.1g, Sugar: 0.2g, Protein: 3.3g

Chocolate Cream Cheese Chaffles

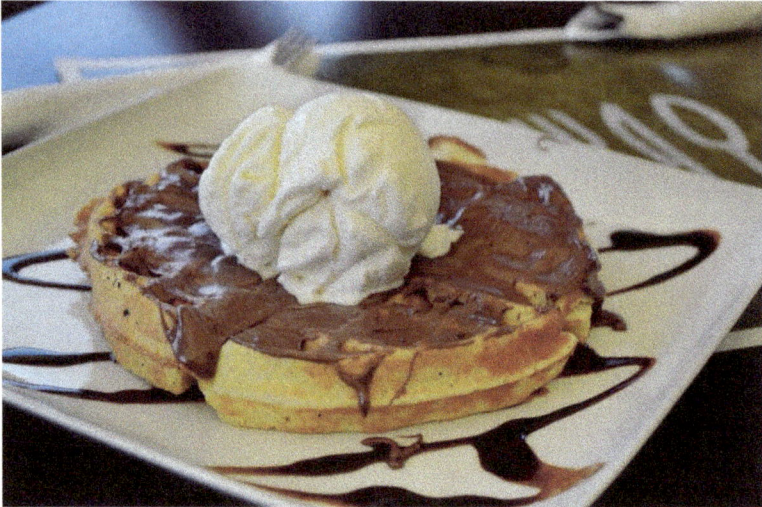

Cooking: 8 Minutes

Servings: 2

Ingredients

- 1 large organic egg, beaten
- 1 ounce of cream cheese, softened
- 1 tbspn sugar-free chocolate syrup
- 1 tbspn Erythritol
- ½ tbspn cacao powder
- ¼ teaspn organic baking powder

- ½ teaspn organic vanilla extract

Directions

- Preheat now a mini waffle iron and then grease it.
- In a bowl, place all ingredients and with a fork, mix well until well combined.
- Place half of the mixture into Preheated waffle iron and cook for about 4 minutes or until golden brown.
- Repeat now with the remaining mixture.
- Serve warm.

Nutrition:

Calories: 103, Net Carb: 4.2g, Fat: 7.7g, Saturated Fat: 4.1g, Carbohydrates: 4g, Dietary Fiber: 0.4g, Sugar: 2gProtein: 4.5g

Colby Jack Chaffles

Cooking: 6 Minutes

Servings: 1

Ingredients

- 2 ounce ofs colby jack cheese, sliced thinly in triangles
- 1 large organic egg, beaten

Directions

1. Preheat now a waffle iron and then grease it.
2. Arrange 1 thin layer of cheese slices in the bottom of the preheated waffle iron.
3. Place the beaten egg on top of the cheese.
4. Now, arrange another layer of cheese slices on top to cover evenly.
5. Cook for about 6 minutes.
6. Serve warm.

Nutrition:

Calories 292, Net Carbs 2.4 g, Total Fat 23 g, Saturated Fat 13.6 g, Cholesterol 236 mg, Sodium 431 mg, Total Carbs 2.4 g, Fiber 0 g, Sugar 0.4 g, Protein 18.3 g

Strawberry Chaffles

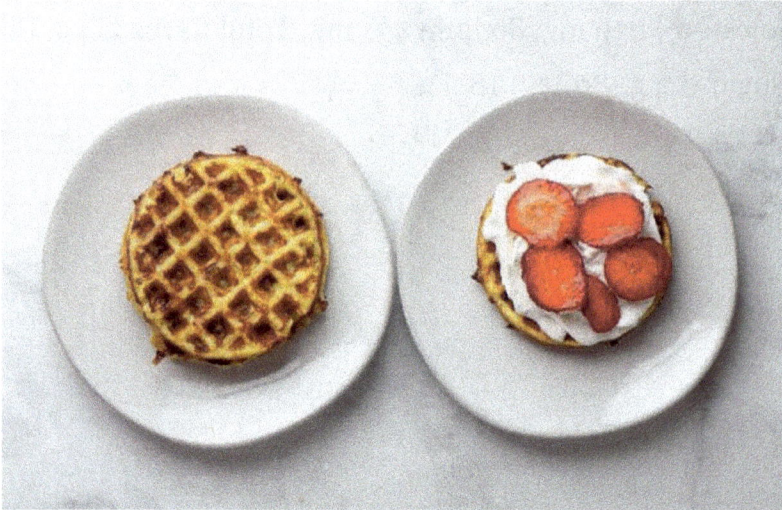

Cooking: 8 Minutes

Servings: 2

Ingredients

- 1 organic egg, beaten
- ¼ cup Mozzarella cheese, shredded
- 1 tbspn cream cheese, softened
- ¼ teaspn organic baking powder
- 1 teaspn organic strawberry extract
- 2 fresh strawberries, hulled and sliced

Directions

- Preheat now a mini waffle iron and then grease it.
- Place all ingredients except strawberry slices and beat in a bowl until well combined.
- Fold in the strawberry slices.
- Place half of the mixture into Preheated waffle iron and cook for about minutes or until golden brown.
- Repeat now with the remaining mixture.
- Serve warm.

Nutrition:

Calories: 69, Net Carb: 1.6g, Fat: 4.6g, Saturated Fat: 2.2g, Carbohydrates: 1.9g, Dietary Fiber: 0.3g, Sugar: 1g, Protein: 4.2g

Mocha Chaffle

Preparation: 8 minutes

Cooking: 9 Minutes

Servings: 3

Ingredients

- 1 organic egg, beaten
- 1 tbspn cacao powder
- 1 tbspn Erythritol
- ¼ teaspn organic baking powder
- 2 tbsps cream cheese, softened
- 1 tbspn mayonnaise
- ¼ teaspn instant coffee powder
- Pinch of salt
- 1 teaspn organic vanilla extract

Directions

1. Preheat now a mini waffle iron and then grease it.
2. In a bowl, place all ingredients and with a fork, Mix well until well combined.

3. Place 1/of the mixture into Preheated waffle iron and cook for about 2½-3 minutes or golden brown.
4. Repeat now with the remaining mixture.
5. Serve warm.

Nutrition:

Calories 202, Fat 6.6, Fiber 5,.4, Carbs 2.9, Protein 9.2

Carrot Chaffle

Preparation: 8 minutes

Cooking: 18 Minutes

Servings: 6

Ingredients

- ¾ cup almond flour
- 1 tbspn walnuts, chopped
- 2 tbsps powdered Erythritol
- 1 teaspn organic baking powder
- ½ teaspn ground cinnamon
- ½ teaspn pumpkin pie spice
- 1 organic egg, beaten
- 2 tbsps heavy whipping cream
- 2 tbsps butter, Melted
- ½ cup carrot, peeled and shredded

Directions

- Preheat now a mini waffle iron and then grease it.

- Place the flour, walnut, Erythritol, cinnamon, baking powder and spices and mix well in a bowl.
- Add the egg, heavy whipping cream and butter and Mix well until well combined.
- Gently, fold in the carrot.
- Add about 3 tbsps of the mixture into Preheated waffle iron and cook for about 2½-3 minutes or golden brown.
- Repeat now with the remaining mixture.
- Serve warm.

Nutrition:

Calories 65, Fat 3.2, Fiber 4.6, Carbs 8.6, Protein 2.6

Yogurt Chaffle

Preparation: 8 minutes

Cooking: 10 Minutes

Servings: 3

Ingredients

- ½ cup shredded Mozzarella
- 1 egg
- 2 Tbsp. ground almonds
- ½ tsp. psyllium husk
- ¼ tsp. baking powder
- 1 Tbsp. yogurt

Directions

- Turn on waffle maker to heat and oil it with cooking spray.
- Whisk eggs in a bowl.
- Add in remaining ingredients except Mozzarella and mix well.
- Add Mozzarella and mix once again. Let it sit for 5 minutes.

- Add batter into each waffle mold.
- Close and cooking for 4-5 minutes.
- Repeat now with remaining batter.

Nutrition:

Calories 304, Fat 8.3, Fiber 4.5, Carbs 1.6, Protein 7

Pumpkin Cake Chaffle with Cream Cheese Frosting

Preparation: 15 minutes

Cooking: 28 minutes

Servings: 4

Ingredients

For the pumpkin chaffles:

- 2 eggs, beaten
- ½ tsp. pumpkin pie spice
- 1 cup finely grated Mozzarella cheese
- 1 tbsp. pumpkin puree

For the cream cheese frosting:

- 2 tbsp. cream cheese, softened
- 2 tbsp. swerve confectioner's sugar
- ½ tsp. vanilla extract

Directions

For the chaffles:

1. Preheat the waffle iron.

2. In a bowl, mix now the egg, pumpkin pie spice, Mozzarella cheese, and pumpkin puree.

3. Open the iron and add a quarter of the mixture. Close and cooking until crispy, 7 minutes.

4. Transfer the chaffle to a plate and make 3 more chaffles with the remaining batter.

For the cream cheese frosting:

5. Add the cream cheese, swerve sugar, and vanilla to a bowl and whisk using an electric mixer until smooth and fluffy.

6. Layer the chaffles one on another but with some frosting spread between the layers. Top with the bit of frosting.

7. Slice and serve.

Nutrition:

Calories 203, Fat 12.3, Fiber 3.1, Carbs 5.9, Protein 4.7

Banana Nut Chaffles

Preparation: 5 minutes

Cooking: 10 Minutes

Servings: 1

Ingredients

- 1 egg
- 1 Tbsp. cream cheese, softened and room temp
- 1 Tbsp. sugar-free cheesecake pudding
- ½ cup Mozzarella cheese
- 1 Tbsp. monk fruit confectioners' sweetener
- ¼ tsp. vanilla extract
- ¼ tsp. banana extract
- toppings of choice

Directions

1. Turn on waffle maker to heat and oil it with cooking spray.
2. Beat egg in a tiny bowl.
3. Add remaining ingredients and Mix well until well incorporated.

4. Add one half of the batter to waffle maker and cooking for min, until golden brown.
5. Remove now chaffle and add the other half of the batter.
6. Top with your optional toppings and serve warm!

Nutrition:

Calories: 246, Total fat: 23g, Protein: 7g, Total carbs: 8g

Chocolaty Chips and Pumpkin Chaffles

Preparation: 5 minutes

Cooking: 12 Minutes

Servings: 3

Ingredients

- 1 organic egg
- 4 teaspns homemade pumpkin puree
- ½ cup Mozzarella cheese, shredded
- 1 tbspn almond flour
- 2 tbsps granulated Erythritol
- ¼ teaspn pumpkin pie spice
- 4 teaspns 70% dark chocolate chips

Directions

- In a bowl, place the egg and pumpkin puree and mix well.
- Add the remaining ingredients except for chocolate chips and Mix well until well combined.
- Gently, fold in the chocolate chips and lemon zest.

96

- Place 1/3 of the mixture into Preheated waffle iron and cooking for about minutes or until golden brown.
- Repeat now with the remaining mixture.
- Serve warm.

Nutrition:

Calories: 229, Total fat: 21g, Protein: 6g, Total carbs: 10g

Finely Knit Chaffles

Preparation: 5 minutes

Cooking: 5 Minutes

Servings: 3

Ingredients

Chocolate Chaffle:

- 2 eggs
- 2 tbsp. cocoa, unsweetened
- 2 tbsp. sweetener
- 2 tbsp. heavy cream
- 2 tsp. coconut flour
- 1/2 tsp. baking powder
- 1 tsp. vanilla

Filling:

- Whipped cream

Directions

1. Pour half of the mixture into the waffle iron. Cooking for 5 minutes.

2. Once ready, carefully remove and repeat now with the remaining chaffle mixture.
3. Allow the cooked chaffles to sit for 3 minutes.
4. Once they have cooled, spread the whipped cream on the chaffles and stack them cream side facing down to form a sandwich.
5. Slice into halves and enjoy.

Nutrition:

Calories: 323, Total fat: 30g, Protein: 9g, Total carbs: 8g

Whipping Cream and Pumpkin Chaffles

Preparation: 8 minutes

Cooking: 12 Minutes

Servings: 2

Ingredients

- 2 organic eggs
- 2 tbsps homemade pumpkin puree
- 2 tbsps heavy whipping cream
- 1 tbspn coconut flour
- 1 tbspn Erythritol
- 1 teaspn pumpkin pie spice
- ½ teaspn organic baking powder
- ½ teaspn organic vanilla extract
- Pinch of salt
- ½ cup Mozzarella cheese, shredded

Directions

- Preheat now a mini waffle iron and then grease it.
- Place all the ingredients except Mozzarella cheese and beat until well combined in a bowl.

- Add the Mozzarella cheese and stir to combine.
- Place half of the mixture into Preheated waffle iron and cooking for about 6 minutes or until golden brown.
- Repeat now with the remaining mixture.
- Serve warm.

Nutrition:

Calories 336, Carbs 3.5, Protein 16.5g, Fat 13.7g, Fiber 2.6g,

Basic Sweet Keto Chaffles

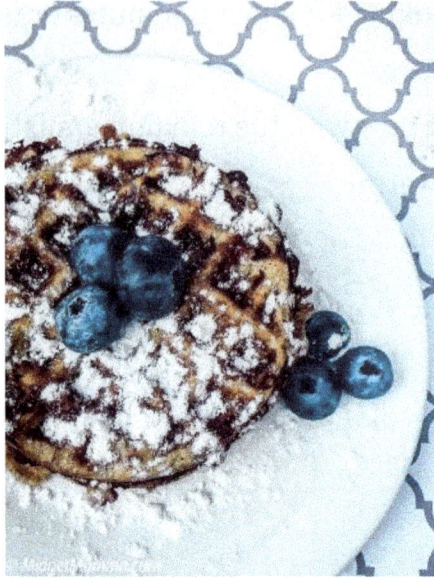

Preparation: 5 minutes

Cooking: 5 Minutes

Servings: 2

Ingredients

- 1 egg
- ½ cup shredded Cheddar cheese

Directions:

1. Turn on waffle maker to heat and oil it with cooking spray.
2. Whisk egg in a bowl until well beaten.
3. Add cheese to the egg and stir well to combine.
4. Pour ½ batter into your waffle maker and close the top. Cooking for 3-5 minutes.
5. Transfer chaffle to a plate and set aside for 2-3 minutes to crisp up.
6. Repeat for remaining batter.

Nutrition:

Calories 127, Fat 5g, Carbs 1g, Protein 20 g

Chocolate & Peanut Butter Chaffle

Preparation: 5 minutes

Cooking: 10 Minutes

Servings: 2

Ingredients

- ½ cup shredded Mozzarella cheese
- 1 Tbsp. cocoa powder
- 2 Tbsp. powdered sweetener
- 2 Tbsp. peanut butter
- ½ tsp. vanilla
- 1 egg
- 2 Tbsp. crushed peanuts
- 2 Tbsp. whipped cream
- ¼ cup sugar-free chocolate syrup

Directions

1. Combine mozzarella, egg, vanilla, peanut butter, cocoa powder, and sweetener in a bowl.
2. Add in peanuts and mix well.
3. Turn on waffle maker and oil it with cooking spray.

4. Pour one half of the batter into waffle maker and cooking for min, then transfer to a plate.
5. Top with whipped cream, peanuts, and sugar-free chocolate syrup.

Nutrition:

Calories 245, Fat 7g, Carbs 23g, Protein 10 g

Butter & Cream Cheese Chaffles

Cooking: 16 Minutes

Servings: 4

Ingredients

- 2 tbsps butter, Melted and cooled
- 2 large organic eggs
- 2 ounce ofs cream cheese, softened
- ¼ cup powdered erythritol
- 1½ teaspns organic vanilla extract
- Pinch of salt
- ¼ cup almond flour
- 2 tbsps coconut flour
- 1 teaspn organic baking powder

Directions

- Preheat now a mini waffle iron and then grease it.
- In a bowl, add the butter and eggs and beat until creamy.
- Add the cream cheese, erythritol, vanilla extract, salt, and beat until well combined.

- Add the flours and baking powder and beat until well combined.
- Place ¼ of the mixture into the preheated waffle iron and cook for about 4 minutes.
- Repeat now with the remaining mixture.
- Serve warm.
- Nutrition: Calories 217, Net Carbs 3.3 g, Total Fat 1g, Saturated Fat 8.8 g, Cholesterol 124 mg, Sodium 173 mg, Total Carbs 6.6 g, Fiber 3.3 g, Sugar 1.2 g, Protein 5.3 g

Cinnamon Chaffles

Cooking: 8 Minutes

Servings: 2

Ingredients

- 1 large organic egg, beaten
- ¾ cup mozzarella cheese, shredded
- ½ tbspn unsalted butter, Melted
- 2 tbsps blanched almond flour
- 2 tbsps erythritol
- ½ teaspn ground cinnamon
- ½ teaspn Psyllium husk powder
- ¼ teaspn organic baking powder
- ½ teaspn organic vanilla extract

Topping:

- 1 teaspn powdered Erythritol
- ¾ teaspn ground cinnamon

Directions

1. Preheat now a waffle iron and then grease it.

2. For chaffles: In a bowl, put all ingredients and mix well until combined with a fork.

3. Place half of the mixture into the Preheated waffle iron and cook for about 5 minutes.

4. Repeat now with the remaining mixture.

5. Meanwhile, in a tiny bowl, mix together the erythritol and cinnamon for topping.

6. Place the chaffles onto serving plates and set aside to cool slightly.

7. Sprinkle with the cinnamon mixture and serve immediately.

Nutrition:

Calories 142, Net Carbs 2.1 g, Total Fat 10.6 g, Saturated Fat 4 g, Cholesterol 106 mg, Sodium 122 mg, Total Carbs 4.1 g, Fiber 2 g, Sugar 0.3 g, Protein 7.7 g

Glazed Chaffles

Cooking: 5 Minutes

Servings: 2

Ingredients

- ½ cup mozzarella shredded cheese
- ⅛ cup cream cheese
- 2 Tbsp unflavored whey protein isolate
- 2 Tbsp swerve confectioners sugar substitute
- ½ tsp baking powder
- ½ tsp vanilla extract
- 1 egg

For the glaze topping:

- 2 Tbsp heavy whipping cream
- 3-4 Tbsp swerve confectioners sugar substitute
- ½ tsp vanilla extract

Directions

1. Turn on waffle maker to heat and oil it with cooking spray.

2. In a microwave-safe bowl, mix mozzarella and cream cheese. Heat at 30 second intervals until melted and fully combined.
3. Add protein, 2 Tbsp sweetener, baking powder to cheese. Knead with hands until well incorporated.
4. Place dough into a mixing bowl and beat in egg and vanilla until a smooth batter form.
5. Put ⅓ of the batter into waffle maker, and cook for 3-min, until golden brown.
6. Repeat until all 3 chaffles are made.
7. Beat glaze ingredients in a bowl and pour over chaffles before serving.

Nutrition:

Carbs: 4 g, Fat: 6 g, Protein: 4 g, Calories: 130

www.ingramcontent.com/pod-product-compliance
Lightning Source LLC
Chambersburg PA
CBHW050748030426
42336CB00012B/1708